MORE CRNA MNEMONICS

125 MORE TIPS, TRICKS, AND
MEMORY CUES TO HELP YOU
KICK-ASS IN CRNA SCHOOL

Chris Mulder, CRNA, MSN

Copyright © 2019 by Kick-Ass Nursing

All rights reserved. This book or any portion thereof may not be reproduced or used in any manner whatsoever without the express written permission of the publisher except for the use of brief quotations in a book review.

The publisher and the author are in no way affiliated with the NCLEX, NBCRNA, or the National Council of State Boards of Nursing (NCSBN). The information in this book is designed to help with fundamental information that may be presented on exams, such as the NCLEX or NBCRNA. However, there is no guarantee of success.

Knowledge and the best practice in this field are continuously changing. As new research and further experience expand our understanding, changes in practice, treatments, and drug therapy may become required or appropriate. Readers are advised to check the most current information provided on the labs and diagnoses that are featured, to verify the recommended doses or formulas, the methods and durations of administration, and contraindications.

It is the responsibility of the practitioner, relying on their own experience and knowledge of the patient, to make diagnoses, to determine dosages and the best treatment for each individual patient, and to take all appropriate safety precautions. To the fullest extent of the law, neither the publisher nor the authors assume any liability for any injury and/or damage to persons or property arising out of or related to any use of the material contained in this book.

Table of Contents

About the Author 11

Introduction 12

Airway 14

    Hypocapnia - Causes 15

    Hypercapnia - Causes 16

    Post-intubation Croup – Risk Factors 17

    One-Lung Ventilation – Absolute Indications 18

    Increase in Dead Space 19

    Trans-tracheal Jet Ventilation - Complications ... 20

    Fiberoptic Bronchoscopy - Contraindications 21

    Pulse Oximetry Artifact – Low Perfusion States .. 22

    PEEP – Potential Disadvantages 23

    Gas Flow Obstruction – Typical Causes 24

Cardiovascular System 25

    Histamine - Cardiovascular Effects 26

    Fat Embolism Syndrome – Symptom Triad 27

    Idiopathic Subaortic Stenosis – Drugs to Avoid ... 28

    Vasospasm – H Therapy 29

    Hypotension During Surgery - Causes 30

    Air Embolism – Treatment 31

    Air Embolism – Detection (Intermediate Sensitivity) 32

    Pulmonary Embolism – Treatment 33

    Hepatic Artery and Portal Vein – Receptors 34

Myocardial Oxygen Demand – Determining Factors 35

Myocardial Oxygen Supply – Determining Factors 36

Aortic Stenosis – Hemodynamic Goals 37

Aortic Insufficiency – Hemodynamic Goals.........38

Valvular Heart Disease – Cardiac Parameters to Monitor..39

Mitral Stenosis – Hemodynamic Goals...............40

Mitral Insufficiency – Hemodynamic Goals 41

Hypertrophic Cardiomyopathy – Hemodynamic Goals 42

Idiopathic Hypertrophic Subaortic Stenosis (IHSS) - Changes that Increase Outflow Obstruction.......43

Pulmonary Artery Catheter – Acceptable Insertion Sites 44

Nervous System *45*

Cerebral Perfusion Pressure (CPP) – Calculation.46

Electroconvulsive Therapy (ECT) – Drugs That Prolong Seizure Activity 47

Increased Intracranial Pressure – Treatments During Anesthesia...48

Controlled Hypotension – Agents Used That Increase Intracranial Pressure (ICP)............49

Cervical Spine – Increased Risk for Potential Instability 50

Trigeminal Nerve – Branches..............................51

Brainstem Medulla – Centers 52

Autonomic Hyperreflexia – Treatment...............53

Intracranial Pressure – IV Agents that Decrease ICP...54

Wake-up Test – Complications 55

Central Pontine Myelinolysis – Precipitating Situations 56

Arnold-Chiari Malformation - Signs and Symptoms 57

Pediatrics/Obstetrics *58*

Persistent Fetal Circulation (Precipitating Factors) 59

Fetal Circulation – 4 things that can compromise it 61

Fetal Circulation – 4 things that can improve utero-placental blood flow 62

Emergence Delirium in Children – Risk Factors...63

Inverted Uterus (During Vaginal Delivery) – Anesthetic Considerations..................................64

Uterine Atony - Anesthetic Management...........65

Fetal Scalp Electrode Placement – Complications 66

Coagulation/ Bleeding Disorders..................... *67*

Disseminated Intravascular Coagulation (DIC) - Treatment 68

Blood Components - Four Most Commonly Administered..69

Thromboelastography (TEG) – Parameters Measured 70

Pharmacology *72*

Nondepolarizing Muscle Relaxants - Classification 73

Clonidine – Clinical Uses 74

Amide Toxicity – Potentiating Agents 75

Local Anesthetics – Ways to Increase Potency 76

Anesthetic Dosing – Agents Dosed by Total Body Weight (in Obese Patients) 77

Statin Therapy – Adverse Effects 78

Glucagon Injection – Systemic Effects 79

Dose-response Curve - Descriptive Characteristics 80

Membrane Diffusion – Dependent Factors 81

Intra-arterial Thiopental Injection – Signs and Symptoms 82

Naloxone – Opioid Actions Easily Reversed 83

Naloxone – Opioid Actions Reversed with Higher Doses 84

Plasma Cholinesterase – Conditions that Diminish its Activity 85

Non-Depolarizing Muscle Relaxants – Potentiating Drugs 86

Antimuscarinics – Administration Reasons 87

Cholinesterase Inhibitors – Quaternary vs Tertiary 88

Class I Antiarrhythmics – Uses 89

Calcium Channel Blockers – Uses 90

Protamine – Adverse Effects 91

Conversions 92

Anaphylactic Reactions – Hypnotics Likely to Cause..93

Anesthesia Basics *94*

Gas Cylinders – Amount Remaining 95

Orbital Muscles...96

Aldrete's Scoring System – Criteria 97

Medical Negligence Action - Elements 98

MRI Contraindications – Implanted Devices.......99

Soda Lime Exhaustion - Indicators 100

Awareness During Anesthesia – Increased Risk 101

Volatile Anesthetics – Renal Changes...............102

Gamma Amino Butyric Acid Type A (GABA$_A$) Receptor – Ligand Binding Sites 103

Heat Loss – Causes (Most to Least) 104

Volatile Inhaled Agents – Trade Names............105

Nitrous Oxide (N$_2$O) – Side Effects 106

Anesthetic Brain Uptake – Dependent Factors .107

Complications / Disorders *108*

Fluid Overload in the TURP Patient – Late Signs 109

Delayed Gastric Emptying – Possible Causes 110

Carcinoid Syndrome – Overproduced Hormonal Mediators...111

Myotonic Dystrophy – Anesthetic Concerns.....112

TURP – Glycine Side Effects 113

Malignant Hyperthermia – Complications After it's Controlled...114

Malignant Hyperthermia – Active Cooling Methods 115

Mandibular Hypoplasia – Associated Congenital Diseases 116

Chronic Alcoholics - Hematologic Abnormalities 117

Bladder Perforation – Signs and Symptoms 118

Lower Esophageal Sphincter Tone – Factors That Decrease 120

Glucose-6-phosphate-dehydrogenase (G6PDH) Deficiency – Drugs to Avoid 121

Duchenne Muscular Dystrophy – Anesthetic Concerns 122

Syndrome of Inappropriate ADH Secretion (SIADH) – Causes 123

Syndrome of Inappropriate ADH Secretion - Treatment 124

Diabetic Autonomic Neuropathy – Anesthetic Concerns 125

Pheochromocytoma – Signs and Symptoms 126

Chronic Renal Failure - Pathophysiological Consequences 127

Complex Regional Pain Syndrome (CRPS) – Signs and Symptoms 128

Prune-belly Syndrome – Congenital Anomalies 129

Burns – Fluid Resuscitation (PA Cath Parameters) 130

Monitoring and Equipment 131

Medical Gas Lines - Common Contaminants 132

Modern Vaporizers – Hazards 133

Proportion-Limiting Systems – Conditions That Can "Fool" Them 134

Required Monitors on the Anesthesia Workstation 135

Regional Anesthesia 136

Stellate Ganglion Blockade (Horner's Syndrome) - Signs and Symptoms 137

Neuraxial Block – Dyspnea Causes 138

Spinal and Epidural Opioids – Side Effects 139

High Spinal Anesthesia – Signs and Symptoms . 140

Retrobulbar Block – Desired Effects 141

Surgical Procedures 142

Mediastinoscopy - Relative Contraindications .. 143

LeFort III Fracture – Important Considerations . 144

Mediastinoscopy – Vessels That Can Be Compressed 145

Strabismus Repair – Anesthetic Concerns 146

Radical Neck Dissection - Intraoperative Complications 147

Pathophysiology 148

Oxyhemoglobin Dissociation Curve - Rightward Shift Causes 149

Adrenal Medulla – Catecholamines Secreted ... 150

Natriuretic Peptides 151

Immunoglobulins 152

Signal Transduction Systems - Components 153

About the Author

My name is Chris Mulder, a full-time nurse anesthetist at a level 1 trauma center in Central Florida. Long before becoming a CRNA, I worked in a tiny cubicle all day in a position that rendered my English degree useless. That only lasted a couple of years before I realized something had to change before I lost my mind. Much to my wife's dismay, I decided to go back to school to get my nursing degree. It wasn't easy, but I made it through. After graduation, I worked as a registered nurse in the medical ICU in a large hospital in Lakeland, FL. A few years later, I applied for Nurse Anesthesia School, and the rest is history!

As I've gone through my years of training and working as a nurse, I've come to realize a few things. The information I was getting in the classroom was difficult to retain and rarely translated to real-world practice. I also found that most nurses took themselves too seriously and were often condescending. That's why I try to keep things a little more light-hearted without all the arrogance.

I know what you're going through. I remember the constant struggle and the sleepless nights. I know the butterflies in the stomach before clinicals and the sinking feeling right before submitting an exam. Stick with me and we'll get through this together. You'll be a CRNA before you know it!

Introduction

Mnemonics can be a great tool to help your brain trigger specific information that you need to know quickly. This tactic can be used for exams, during questioning by instructors, or in your everyday clinical practice. It should be noted that memory tricks like these should not be thought of as a replacement for knowledge of the subject. You first need to understand the core concepts before the mnemonics will be able to help.

The good news is that once you have a grasp on the material you are trying to learn, mnemonics can make your life much easier. This is especially true in the world of anesthesia. There are thousands of diagnoses, labs, medications, symptoms, and treatments. Even after you learn something new, it is easy to get things mixed up.

The idea here isn't to read this entire book to try to remember every single mnemonic. You'll drive yourself crazy that way. Rather, it is meant to be used as a guide as you progress through your anesthesia education and even as you begin your career as a provider.

When you start to cover a specific topic in school, come back to this book and see if there is a mnemonic for it. If you've graduated and there is something you just can't seem to remember, see if we have something that will help. This way, you will be learning as you go, and will be less likely to get the mnemonics mixed up.

Also, keep in mind that mnemonics will never have all the possible information for a specific topic. Only the most important things are covered, and sometimes items are left out for the sake of the mnemonic. It would be impossible to condense a 50-page chapter on the airway into a few words.

Some of these mnemonic devices are commonly known and I have used them myself many times. However, the majority of them are original creations by yours truly. Some of them may sound strange and funny. But this is a good thing! Those are the ones you are more likely to remember.

If something in this book just doesn't seem to be working for you, try to come up with your own mnemonic for that subject. It's not hard. Just try putting letters together to make up words or sentences that you can draw from when the time comes.

If you have any questions about anything in this book, please feel free to email me at contact@kickassnursing.com. Visit us on our web site at www.kickassnursing.com and check out the blog and our other books, such as the original CRNA Mnemonics or Survive CRNA School, to help you get through. Enjoy the mnemonics!

Airway

Hypocapnia - Causes

Hyper CHAD

Hyperventilation

Cold
Hypotension
Anesthesia
Dead space ventilation decreased

Hypocapnia is when the CO2 levels in the body fall to below normal levels and can be caused by many factors. Hyperventilation is a common culprit, whether this be by means of voluntary or mechanical ventilation. It can also be the result of decreased CO2 production (hypothermia, deep anesthesia, hypotension) and decreased dead space ventilation (decreased PEEP, decreased rebreathing, etc). It may be seen in hypothermia or during periods of hypotension. By far the most common cause of hypocapnia is hyperventilation by mechanical means.

Hypercapnia - Causes

CHI

CO2 absorber exhausted
Hypoventilation
Increased dead space ventilation

Hypercapnia is the increase of carbon dioxide in the body above normal levels. Anything that produces more CO2 can be the cause of hypercapnia. For example, you might see it when the CO2 absorber is exhausted, during hypoventilation (depression of ventilation by drugs such as opioids), or when there is an increase in dead space ventilation.

Post-intubation Croup – Risk Factors

HELPER

Head and neck procedures
Early childhood (14 years or less)
Large endotracheal tube
Prolonged surgery
Excessive movement of the endotracheal tube
Repeated intubation attempts

Croup in the post-surgical patient who was intubated is caused by tracheal or glottic edema. There are many things that may play a role, increasing the risk. For example, any procedure that is done in the head and neck area could be the culprit. A large endotracheal tube, excessive movement of the tube, or repeated intubation attempts will all cause irritation to the trachea and glottic opening. Prolonged surgery may also increase the risk for post-intubation croup, as does being a child. Sometimes, it is just going to happen regardless of any precautions, but try to be aware of the common risk factors and adjust appropriately.

One-Lung Ventilation – Absolute Indications

Confine **S**ingle **L**ung **F**irst

Cysts or unilateral bullae
Secretions in one lung
Lavage
Fistula

Although one-lung ventilation is usually voluntary to facilitate surgery, it is sometimes necessary due to other factors. For example, if a patient has cysts or bullae on one side, they may rupture during positive pressure ventilation. Also, contamination of both lungs could be deadly, so blood or infectious secretions in one lung indicates the need for lung isolation. If bronchopulmonary lavage is being done, it is needed to prevent spilling over of fluid to the nondependent lung. Lastly, a bronchopleural fistula or a bronchocutaneous fistula mandates one-lung ventilation.

Increase in Dead Space

APPLE

Age
Positive-pressure ventilation
Pulmonary embolism
Lung disease
Extension of Neck/Jaw

Dead space is the portion of air that is inhaled (or delivered), but doesn't participate in gas exchange. This could be caused by many things, and is increased by age, positive-pressure ventilation, pulmonary embolism, lung disease, and extension of the neck and jaw. Another common thing that increases dead space is the breathing circuit. The longer the circuit, the more dead space there is. This air basically gets wasted, doing neither harm nor good.

Trans-tracheal Jet Ventilation - Complications

SAME BED

Subcutaneous emphysema
Arterial perforation
Mediastinal emphysema
Exhalation difficulty

Barotrauma
Esophageal puncture
Damage to tracheal mucosa

Trans-tracheal jet ventilation is sometimes used when difficult airways are expected or in certain surgical procedures when very low tidal volumes are needed. It is not very common, but it's important to know the potential complications when you are faced with this challenge. Barotrauma can result in pneumothorax, while air can also enter as subcutaneous emphysema or mediastinal emphysema. Arterial perforation and damage to the tracheal mucosa is a potential complication, as is esophageal puncture, which will result in bleeding and hemoptysis.

Fiberoptic Bronchoscopy - Contraindications

BLUSH

Bleeding
Local Anesthetic Allergy
Unable to Cooperate
Secretions
Hypoxia

While fiberoptic bronchoscopy may be useful in many situations, it is also contraindicated under certain circumstances. If a patient is bleeding from any part of the airway and is not resolved with suction, you might want to put the scope down. Hypoxia and heavy airway secretions (even after suction and antisialagogues) are also a contraindication. For an awake fiberoptic attempt, the patient should be able to cooperate and receive local anesthesia. If not, you should probably consider another way.

Pulse Oximetry Artifact – Low Perfusion States

HAIL

Hypothermia
Anemia
Increased systemic vascular resistance
Low cardiac output

Pulse oximetry artifact can be caused by a few different things, including electrical interference, moving/shaking, malfunction, and low perfusion states. Hypothermia, anemia, increased systemic vascular resistance, and low cardiac output are all examples of low perfusion states that may cause pulse oximetry artifact. One way to get a better reading on the monitor is to place the probe in a better perfused area, such as the earlobe or forehead.

PEEP – Potential Disadvantages

RIP

Redistribution of pulmonary blood flow
Increased extravascular lung water
Pulmonary barotrauma

PEEP is positive end-expiratory pressure, something that can be very beneficial for certain patient populations and in certain situations. But it can have potential disadvantages also. PEEP can cause redistribution of pulmonary blood flow from the core to the periphery. It may also cause increased extravascular lung water, which is the fluid that accumulates in the alveolar and interstitial spaces. Another issue could be pulmonary barotrauma if the PEEP and tidal volume are too much for the patient's lungs.

Gas Flow Obstruction – Typical Causes

BECK

Blood or secretions in the ETT
Expiratory valve malfunction
Cuff herniation
Kinking of the ETT

There aren't many things more annoying than hearing a high-pressure alarm from the ventilator, and can be quite nerve racking when you can't figure out the source of the problem. There may be several reasons for gas flow obstruction, but some common ones include kinking of the ET tube, blood/secretions in the ET tube, expiratory valve malfunction, and cuff herniation. Cuff herniation is possible if it is overinflated (if it doesn't rupture), going over the ET tube, effectively blocking it. You would also get the high-pressure alarm if the patient is coughing or pushing against the vent, having a bronchospasm, or if a mucous plug is present.

Cardio-vascular System

Histamine - Cardiovascular Effects

CRIES

Chronotropic
Relaxes smooth muscles
Inotropic
Edema
Stimulates adrenal medulla

Histamine has many effects in the body, and the cardiovascular system is no different. When it's released, either from natural reasons or from medications, the heart rate increases (chronotropic) and the smooth muscles of arterioles and small blood vessels relax (hypotension). It also causes edema by increasing capillary permeability, as well as stimulating the adrenal medulla to release catecholamines.

Fat Embolism Syndrome – Symptom Triad

Come **H**elp **P**lease

Confusion
Hypoxemia
Petechiae

Fat embolism syndrome is a potential complication with fractures or during orthopedic surgery. Three of the most common symptoms are hypoxemia, petechia, and confusion or respiratory distress (in awake patients). If these three symptoms present, along with orthopedic involvement, then it would be wise to suspect fat embolism syndrome.

Idiopathic Subaortic Stenosis – Drugs to Avoid

Don't **P**oke **B**oob **V**eins

Diuretics
Positive inotropes
Beta adrenergic agonists
Vasodilators

Idiopathic subaortic stenosis is a type of left ventricular outflow obstruction. Certain medications should be avoided in patients with this condition, as they can sometimes worsen the obstruction. These agents include diuretics, beta adrenergic agonists, positive inotropes (calcium, digitalis), and vasodilators (nitroprusside, nitroglycerine). Sorry for the randomness of this mnemonic, but I'll bet you won't forget Don't Poke Boob Veins.

Vasospasm – H Therapy

Hypervolemia
Hemodilution
Hypertension

When a patient is having a vasospasm, 'H' therapy can be a successful treatment. Colloids and Crystalloids should be given aggressively to keep the CVP higher than 10 mmHg or the PCWP 12-20 mmHg. Be careful not to put the patient into congestive heart failure. They should also be hemodiluted to a hematocrit of around 33 percent. This can help to balance viscosity and oxygen-carrying capacity. Hypertension should also be a goal by using agents such as dopamine, phenylephrine, and dobutamine. The systolic blood pressure should be maintained around 160-200 mmHg.

Hypotension During Surgery - Causes

CVS Drugs

Contractility (Decreased)
Venous return (Preload – Decreased)
Systemic vascular resistance (Decreased)
Dysrhythmias

Hypotension is a common occurrence while a patient is under anesthesia. While we know that a bleeding patient or dehydrated patient will drop their blood pressure, you should know the basic physiologic reasons. Common causes include decreased contractility, decreased systemic vascular resistance, and dysrhythmias. A decreased preload will also cause hypotension.

Air Embolism – Treatment

DARES

Durant Maneuver
Aspiration
Release Pneumoperitoneum
Eliminate Nitrous Oxide
Stop Insufflation

Air embolism during surgery is a very dangerous thing that must be acted upon quickly. Make the surgeon aware of the situation, have them stop the insufflation, and release the peritoneum. If you have nitrous oxide running, turn it off. If the patient has a central line, you can try aspirating the air from the right atrium. You can also try repositioning, using the Durant Maneuver, putting the patient in a left-lateral tilt and Trendelenburg.

Air Embolism – Detection (Intermediate Sensitivity)

Put some **PEP** in your step

Pulmonary artery pressure
End-tidal CO2
PaO2

Early treatment of air embolism is extremely important. But before treatment can be started, the problem must first be identified. The patient will have a decreased PaO2, decreased end-tidal CO2, and an elevated pulmonary artery pressure. These forms of detection are considered to be intermediate sensitivity.

Pulmonary Embolism – Treatment

O SHIT

Oxygen

Support cardiovascular function
Heparin
Intubate if necessary
Treat hypotension

If you're ever faced with the terrifying situation of an intraoperative pulmonary embolism, it is important to know how to respond quickly. The first thing is to treat the symptoms that are presenting in the moment and if it's a big PE, making sure they don't die. You might just be in ACLS mode at this point. In general, though, you will want to give more oxygen and intubate if necessary, treat hypotension and support cardiovascular function, and start the patient on anticoagulation once stable.

Hepatic Artery and Portal Vein – Receptors

Hepatic Artery:

ABCD

Alpha-1 (vasoconstriction)
Beta-2 (vasodilation)
Cholinergic (vasodilation)
D1 (vasodilation)

Portal Vein:

AD

Alpha-1 (vasoconstriction)
D1 (vasodilation)

In the liver, the hepatic artery and portal vein have receptors that each function to cause either vasodilation or vasoconstriction, among other things. Alpha-1 and D1 receptors can be found on both the hepatic artery and portal vein. Alpha-1 causes vasoconstriction, while D1 causes vasodilation. Beta-2 receptors and cholinergic receptors are found on the hepatic artery and they both cause vasodilation.

Myocardial Oxygen Demand – Determining Factors

CHAP

Contractility
Heart rate
Afterload
Preload

Myocardial oxygen demand is increased when more of it is being used. The factors that determine this include contractility, heart rate, afterload, and preload. Afterload is the systolic wall tension, while preload is the diastolic wall tension. When one of these factors is increased, the myocardial oxygen consumption is also increased, thereby increasing myocardial oxygen demand. On the other hand, when one of these factors is decreased, oxygen consumption is also decreased, thereby decreasing myocardial oxygen demand.

Myocardial Oxygen Supply – Determining Factors

HALO

Heart Rate
Aortic Diastolic Pressure
Left Ventricular End-diastolic Pressure
Oxygen Content/**O**xygen Extraction

Myocardial oxygen supply is determined by several factors. A high heart rate could lower perfusion because of the decrease in the diastole time (when coronary blood flow occurs). If the aortic diastolic pressure is low, then perfusion pressure is low. A high left ventricular end-diastolic pressure could decrease flow by compressing the subendocardium. Lastly, myocardial oxygen supply is determined by the obvious: the amount of oxygen content in arterial blood and the amount of oxygen being extracted.

Aortic Stenosis – Hemodynamic Goals

Silly Full Time RN

Slow (low heart rate)
Full (maintained or increased preload)
Tight (maintained or increased afterload - SVR)
Regular (maintain sinus rhythm)
Not too strong (maintain contractility).

A major goal with aortic stenosis patients is to not let the heart rate increase. You'll also want to maintain or even increase the preload (Full), maintain or increase the afterload (Tight), keep them in normal sinus rhythm (Regular), and maintain the contractility (Not too strong). AS: Always Slow.

Aortic Insufficiency – Hemodynamic Goals

Fat, Fake, Farting RN

Fast (high heart rate)
Full (increase preload)
Forward (decrease afterload)
Regular (maintain sinus rhythm)
Not too strong (maintain contractility)

When you are encountered with a patient who has aortic insufficiency, remember first and foremost to keep the heart rate up (Fast). You should also make it a goal to increase the preload (Full), decrease the afterload (Forward), keep them in normal sinus rhythm (Regular), and maintain the contractility (Not too strong). AI: Always Increased.

Valvular Heart Disease – Cardiac Parameters to Monitor

PARCH

Preload
Afterload (determined by SVR)
Rhythm
Contractility
Heart rate

While taking care of a patient who has existing valvular heart disease, there are several cardiac parameters that should be monitored, especially while under anesthesia. These monitors include preload, afterload, rhythm, contractility, and heart rate.

Mitral Stenosis – Hemodynamic Goals

Silly **N**ight **N**urse **RN**

Slow (low heart rate)
Not too full (maintained preload)
Not too tight (maintained afterload (SVR)
Regular (maintain sinus rhythm)
Not too strong (maintained contractility)

Patients with mitral stenosis will greatly appreciate it if you can keep their heart rate low (Slow). You should also make it a goal to maintain the preload (Not too full), maintain the afterload (Not too tight), maintain the contractility (Not too strong), and keep them in normal sinus rhythm (Regular). MS: Make Slow.

Mitral Insufficiency – Hemodynamic Goals

Funny **N**urse **F**orgot **R**eggie's **M**eds

Fast (increase heart rate)
Not too full (maintain to slightly increase preload)
Forward (decrease afterload)
Regular (maintain normal sinus rhythm)
Maintain contractility

It's important to consider many hemodynamic goals when it comes to patients with mitral insufficiency. While it's vital to keep their heart rate up (Fast), don't forget to maintain or even increase the preload (Not too full), decrease the afterload (Forward), maintain the contractility, and keep them in normal sinus rhythm (Regular). Try to avoid anything that would cause an increase in pulmonary vascular resistance. MI: Myocardial Increase.

Hypertrophic Cardiomyopathy – Hemodynamic Goals

My Face Turns Red Nightly

Maintain normal heart rate
Full (increased preload)
Tight (increased afterload)
Regular (normal sinus rhythm is crucial)
Not too strong (slightly depressed myocardial contractility)

Hypertrophic cardiomyopathy causes the heart to become thicker, thereby making it more difficult to pump blood through. For these patients, it's important to try to maintain a normal heart rate, keep the preload higher (Full), increase the afterload (Tight), and somewhat depressed contractility (Not too strong).

Idiopathic Hypertrophic Subaortic Stenosis (IHSS) - Changes that Increase Outflow Obstruction

II DD CHAP

Increased **C**ontractility
Increased **H**eart rate
Decreased **A**fterload
Decreased **P**reload

Idiopathic hypertrophic subaortic stenosis causes the left ventricle to become hypertrophied, narrowing the outflow tract and impeding left ventricle ejection. This can be made worse by increased contractility, increased heart rate, decreased afterload, and decreased preload. For these patients, try to maintain or slightly decrease contractility, decrease the heart rate, increase the afterload, and increase the preload.

Pulmonary Artery Catheter – Acceptable Insertion Sites

(In order of ease of insertion)

FEARS

Femoral veins.
External jugular
Antecubital—preferably basilic
Right internal jugular
Subclavian

When inserting a pulmonary artery catheter, several sites are acceptable for insertion. The femoral vein is the easiest place to put it, followed by the external jugular vein, the antecubital vein (basilic is preferred), the right internal jugular vein, and the subclavian vein. The left internal jugular vein should not be used as a site of insertion due to the increased incidence of possible complications.

Nervous System

Cerebral Perfusion Pressure (CPP) – Calculation

CPP = **M**AP – **I**CP

Candy = **M**ike – **I**ke

If you know the mean arterial pressure and the intracranial pressure, then you can easily figure out what the cerebral perfusion pressure is. Simply subtract the ICP from the MAP. This can also work in other ways. For example, you can figure out the MAP if you know what the CPP and the ICP is. You can also figure out what the ICP is if you know the CPP and the MAP. However, there is an exception to this rule. If the right atrial pressure (RAP) is abnormally elevated and higher than the intracranial pressure (ICP), then the cerebral perfusion pressure (CPP) = MAP-RAP, rather than MAP-ICP.

Electroconvulsive Therapy (ECT) – Drugs That Prolong Seizure Activity

CAKE

Caffeine, **C**lozapine
Aminophylline, **A**lfentanil
Ketamine
Etomidate

Electroconvulsive Therapy is commonly used to treat depression and other psychological issues, such as bipolar disorder. While we want these patients to be asleep and comfortable, we don't want to use medications that may depress seizure activity. In fact, some of the medications can actually prolong seizure activity. These include caffeine, clozapine, aminophylline, alfentanil, ketamine, and etomidate. These procedures are relatively short and typically do not require an endotracheal tube.

Increased Intracranial Pressure – Treatments During Anesthesia

CRASHED

Cerebral Vasoconstrictor/**C**ool the Patient
Restrict Fluids
Avoid Hypertension
Steroid
Hyperventilate
Elevate the Head
Dehydrate the Brain

The anesthetist has many options to treat increased intracranial pressure. A cerebral vasoconstrictor may be used, such as etomidate, thiopental, or Propofol. You might consider cooling the patient to 34 degrees Celsius, as this can help to protect the brain while surgery is going on. Fluids should be restricted as the patient's condition allows, and hypertension should be avoided. The brain can be dehydrated by using mannitol or Lasix. Hyperventilation should help by causing more cerebral vasoconstriction, while elevating the head of the bed to 30 degrees should help cerebral venous drainage. Steroids, such as dexamethasone, may be helpful in decreasing localized edema that is surrounding tumors.

Controlled Hypotension – Agents Used That Increase Intracranial Pressure (ICP)

NASH

Nitroglycerin
Adenosine
Sodium nitroprusside
Hydralazine

Sometimes, it's necessary to keep the patient's blood pressure lower in certain circumstances, often to prevent excessive bleeding. To accomplish this, controlled hypotension may be done. But the anesthesia provider should be aware of the ramifications of the medications given to accomplish this. Nitroglycerin, Adenosine, Sodium nitroprusside, and Hydralazine can all increase intracranial pressure while lowering the blood pressure. This is especially important to know because controlled hypotension is often done during neurological procedures.

Cervical Spine – Increased Risk for Potential Instability

NAILS

Neck pain
Any neurological signs or symptoms
Intoxication
Loss of consciousness at the scene
Severe distracting pain

When dealing with a trauma, ruling out a cervical spine injury is extremely important. But before you can get the patient to radiology to confirm anything, it would be a good idea to look at their symptoms. If they are having neck pain, you should investigate further. Are they intoxicated or are there any other neurological signs or symptoms? Is their pain severe and distracting? Was their loss of consciousness at the scene? All of these things make the patient at a greater risk for cervical spine instability.

Trigeminal Nerve – Branches

MOM

Maxillary
Ophthalmic
Mandibular

The trigeminal nerve, which just so happens to be cranial nerve V, provides sensory innervation to the region of the face. The three branches of the trigeminal nerve include the maxillary, ophthalmic, and mandibular. The mandibular branch provides both motor and sensory innervation, while the maxillary and ophthalmic branches provide only sensory innervation.

Brainstem Medulla – Centers

CVS **C**opy**R**ight

Coughing
Vomiting
Swallowing

Cardiovascular
Respiratory

The brainstem consists of the pons, the midbrain, and the medulla oblongata. The medulla is the lower part of the brainstem connected to the spinal cord. It is responsible for coughing, vomiting, sneezing, and swallowing. It is also the portion of the brain that controls the cardiovascular and respiratory systems. Therefore, the medulla is what takes care of blood pressure, heart rate, and breathing.

Autonomic Hyperreflexia – Treatment

DVR

Deepening Anesthesia
Vasodilator
Removal of Stimulus

Autonomic hyperreflexia, also known as autonomic dysreflexia, typically happens with patients who have a spinal cord injury at T7 or above. Patients with other disorders, such as Guillain-Barré syndrome and multiple sclerosis, could also be susceptible. When these patients come in contact with certain stimuli, the nervous system may overreact, causing hypertension and tachycardia at first, with an extreme vagal response likely to follow shortly after. A common stimulus for this response is overdistension of the bladder.

If your patient has this type of response during surgery, the first step that has the highest chance of stopping it is to remove the stimulus causing it. If the bladder is distended, insert a catheter to drain it. If the surgeon is irrigating the bladder for a urology procedure, have them release some of the pressure. You can also try deepening the anesthesia, so the response isn't quite as profound. A vasodilator may be used if it continues (i.e. sodium nitroprusside).

Intracranial Pressure – IV Agents that Decrease ICP

BEBOP

Benzodiazepines
Etomidate
Barbiturates
Opioids
Propofol

Whether intended or not, several medications that we give have the ability to decrease intracranial pressure. These include benzodiazepines, such as versed, etomidate, and Propofol. It also happens with barbiturates, such as phenobarbital, and opioids, such as morphine.

Wake-up Test – Complications

DREAMS

Dislodgement of Instrumentation
Recall
Extubation
Air Embolus
Myocardial Ischemia
Self-injury

Wake-up tests are used in some neurosurgical cases to see if the patient is still neurologically intact during or after a critical point. When this is done, several complications are possible. For instance, any instrumentation the surgeon has in place may become dislodged. Although rare, the patient may have recall after the surgery is complete. If they move too much, they could possibly extubate themselves or cause accidental injury. If the patient takes a deep breath, they could get an air embolus from open venous sinuses.

Central Pontine Myelinolysis – Precipitating Situations

HOT

Head injury
Orthotopic liver transplantation
TURP syndrome

Central pontine myelinolysis is a neurological problem that usually happens after correction of hyponatremia. When it is corrected too rapidly with hypertonic saline, it can damage the myelin sheath of the brainstem (pons portion) nerve cells. These patients will have an altered level of consciousness, with eventual difficulty speaking and swallowing. If untreated, the patients can become paralyzed, "locked-in," and eventually die. Head injury, TURP syndrome, and orthotopic liver transplantation can all cause hyponatremia. Therefore, they are precipitating situations that could lead to CPM if the low sodium is treated too quickly.

Arnold-Chiari Malformation - Signs and Symptoms

ARDS

Apneic episodes
Recurrent aspiration
Difficulty swallowing
Stridor

Arnold-Chiari malformation is a condition that consists of the herniation of the cerebellar tonsils through the foramen magnum, often compressing the brainstem also. Common symptoms include episodes of apnea, recurrent aspiration, dysphagia, and stridor. These patients may also have frequent headaches, vomiting, neck pain, tinnitus, neuropathies, and scoliosis, among others.

Pediatrics/Obstetrics

Persistent Fetal Circulation (Precipitating Factors)

Have **A** **H**elpful **P**ediatrician

Hypoxemia
Acidosis
Hypothermia
Pneumonia

You may recall that babies in utero have a different circulatory pattern. They are connected to the mother's blood by way of the umbilical cord. Blood comes through the umbilical cord and the ductus venosus shunts the oxygenated blood away from the liver and in the direction of the heart. This blood then goes through the inferior vena cava (IVC) into the right atrium. This blood then enters the left atrium via the foramen ovale, bypassing the lungs. The ductus arteriosus also shunts blood away from the lungs, into the aorta. This mixed blood then travels through the rest of the fetal body before going back to the placenta.

Once the baby is born, the umbilical cord gets clamped, interrupting this fetal blood flow. The baby starts to breathe and the lungs expand. The blood pressure increases and pulmonary pressures decrease, eventually leading to the closure of the foramen ovale and ductus arteriosus.

In persistent fetal circulation, there is increased pulmonary vascular resistance and right-to-left shunting, thereby preventing the normal circulatory changes from taking place. This can be common in preterm infants and infants with metabolic abnormalities such as sepsis, congenital diaphragmatic hernia, meconium aspiration, hypothermia, and asphyxia.

Fetal Circulation – 4 things that can compromise it

HEAL

Hypoxemia (maternal)
Excessive uterine activity
Aortocaval compression
Low blood pressure (maternal)

Fetal Circulation – 4 things that can improve utero-placental blood flow

FOME (Fear Of Missing Everything)

Fluids
Oxytocin infusion adjustment
Maternal position changes (to avoid aortocaval compression)
Ephedrine

Emergence Delirium in Children – Risk Factors

CAT CRAP

Child Temperament
Age
Type of Surgery

Characteristic of anesthetic
Rapid Emergence
Adjunct Medication
Preoperative Anxiety

Emergence delirium can happen with any child after receiving anesthesia. But certain characteristics may point to an increased likelihood of it happening. Children under five years old are more likely to experience emergence delirium, as are those with a poor temperament (poor socialization, difficulty adapting). It is more common after ophthalmologic and otolaryngologic surgeries and when adjunct medications, such as opioids, are used. You may also see it when the emergence from anesthesia is done rapidly or when the child is very anxious in pre-op. In most cases of emergence delirium, the child was anxious in the pre-operative area.

Inverted Uterus (During Vaginal Delivery) – Anesthetic Considerations

Baby **GROWL**

Blood Ready

General Anesthesia
Rapid Sequence Induction
Oxygen
Warm Fluids
Large Bore Catheters

An inverted uterus during vaginal delivery is a serious issue that must be taken care of quickly. For surgery, there are some anesthetic considerations that must be taken when you go back to the OR. The plan should include general anesthesia with a volatile anesthetic using rapid sequence induction. Once the ET tube is secured, place an OG tube to suction gastric contents. Have blood readily available and be prepared to give a lot of fluid through large bore IVs. Make sure the fluids are warmed to prevent hypothermia.

Uterine Atony - Anesthetic Management

V BOOT

Vital Signs

Blood Replacement
Oxygen
Oxytocin
Trendelenburg

Uterine tone and contraction are required to stop the bleeding after the birth of the baby. Uterine atony is when there is a loss of tone after delivery. This can be managed with medications, such as oxytocin, methergine, and hemabate. Blood loss should be replaced by crystalloids or colloids, followed by blood if necessary. You can try placing the patient in the Trendelenburg position and give oxygen by face mask. Monitor the vital sign closely, including central venous pressure to monitor fluid status if a central line is available.

Fetal Scalp Electrode Placement – Complications

SELLS

Sepsis
Ecchymoses
Lacerations
Leakage of cerebrospinal fluid
Scalp abscesses

A fetal scalp electrode is a wire that is used to closely and reliably monitor variability of fetal heart rate. Common complications of this practice include sepsis, ecchymosis, laceration, and leakage of CSF. However, the most common problem that happens is abscess on the scalp. There may also be complications for the mother, including damage to the vagina wall (i.e. laceration).

Coagulation/ Bleeding Disorders

Disseminated Intravascular Coagulation (DIC) - Treatment

People **C**ry **E**very **F**riday

Platelets
Cryoprecipitate
Eliminate the underlying cause
Fresh-frozen plasma

Disseminated Intravascular Coagulation (DIC) happens when excessive clotting is caused by some injury or disease. The clotting proteins may eventually get depleted, leading to excessive bleeding and organ injury. Treatment may include blood products, such as platelets, cryoprecipitate, and fresh-frozen plasma. Elimination of the underlying cause is paramount to recovery, but you may find yourself treating the symptoms as they come until that happens.

Blood Components - Four Most Commonly Administered

Poor **P**eople **Cry** **F**requently

Packed red blood cells
Platelet concentrates
Cryoprecipitate
Fresh frozen plasma

As anesthesia providers, we administer many types of blood components. But the four most common are packed red blood cells, platelets, cryoprecipitate, and fresh frozen plasma. These are some of the types of questions you may see on boards.

Thromboelastography (TEG) – Parameters Measured

L MARK

LY30 (Clot Lysis)

MA (Maximum Amplitude)
Alpha angle (α)
R (Reaction Time)
K (Clot Formation Time)

Thromboelastography (TEG) is a good measurement to determine how well platelets are functioning, providing information on the quality, rather than just a number. It can be helpful in directing blood transfusion during certain surgeries, such as major trauma, cardiac, and liver transplantation. The five parameters that are monitored in a TEG include clot lysis, maximum amplitude, alpha angle, reaction time, and clot formation time.

The LY30 represents fibrinolysis as an equation, shown as a percent decrease in amplitude after maximum amplitude. MA represents maximum amplitude, the point at which the fibrin clot is the strongest. The alpha angle represents how quickly the clot forms. The reaction time (R) represents the amount of time it takes for the clot to begin to form. Finally, the clot formation time (K) represents the amount of time it takes for the clot to reach a specific strength, based on thrombin and platelet activation.

Pharmacology

Nondepolarizing Muscle Relaxants - Classification

Benzylisoquinoliniums

"curium"

Miva**curium**
Atra**curium**
Cisatra**curium**
Doxa**curium**
d-tubocurarine (exception – no longer used)
Metocurine (exception – no longer used)

Steroid Derivatives

"curonium"

Ve**curonium**
Ro**curonium**
Pan**curonium**
Pipe**curonium**

Clonidine – Clinical Uses

MOP HANDS

Myocardial ischemia protection
Opioid withdrawal
Preanesthetic medication

Hypertension
Adjunct to regional anesthesia
Neuraxial Analgesia
Diagnose pheochromocytoma
Shivering

Clonidine is an alpha-2 agonist, much like precedex, commonly used for sedation and hypertension. But it can also be useful for other things, such as myocardial ischemia protection in the intraoperative period, as a preanesthetic medication, an adjunct to regional anesthesia, and in spinals and epidurals. It can be helpful in patients who are withdrawing from opioids, taking much of the edge off and decreasing the withdrawal time for many of them. Clonidine is also helpful for shivering, which may be good postoperatively, by inhibiting thermoregulatory vasoconstriction. Finally, it can be an aid in diagnosing pheochromocytoma with the clonidine suppression test. When clonidine is given, catecholamine production is usually decreased. If this doesn't happen, then there is a high likelihood of pheochromocytoma.

Amide Toxicity – Potentiating Agents

Can't **P**rocess **A**mides

Cimetidine
Propranolol
Anesthetic gases

When we're talking about amide toxicity, we're talking about inhibition of our old friend, the cytochrome P450 system. Cimetidine, Propranolol, and volatile anesthetics are all examples of agents that potentiate amide toxicity. They inhibit the cytochrome P450 system, thereby decreasing the clearance of amides, causing buildup.

Local Anesthetics – Ways to Increase Potency

Help **C**rnas **E**levate **L**ocals

Halide to the aromatic ring
Carbon atoms
Ester linkage
Large alkyl group on the tertiary amide nitrogen

Lipid solubility and potency may be increased by adding things chemically. Try to stay awake while we go through a little chemistry. One way to increase potency is by adding a halide to the aromatic benzene ring. Examples of halides are chloride ions, bromide ions, etc. You can also add carbon atoms or an ester linkage. Lastly, you can add a large alkyl group to the tertiary amide nitrogen.

Anesthetic Dosing – Agents Dosed by Total Body Weight (in Obese Patients)

No **S**kinny **P**eople **D**oses

Neostigmine
Succinylcholine
Propofol
Dexmedetomidine

Some medications should be dosed by ideal body weight, based on the person's height. But some drugs that we give in anesthesia must be based on total body weight, taking every kilogram into account. Some of the medications include neostigmine, succinylcholine, Precedex, and Propofol (as a maintenance dose).

Statin Therapy – Adverse Effects

RICH GM

Rash
Increased liver enzymes
CNS dysfunction
Headache

Gastrointestinal distress
Muscle weakness

Although statin drugs are great for treating hyperlipidemia, they are not without problems. Some common adverse effects include rash, headache, gastrointestinal distress, increased liver enzymes, and hepatotoxicity. They may also cause neurological issues, such as severe depression, and muscle weakness or myalgia. A major concern is myopathy and the resulting rhabdomyolysis, which may eventually lead to death.

Glucagon Injection – Systemic Effects

RIP

Relaxes gastrointestinal smooth muscle
Increases myocardial contractility
Promotes glycogenolysis

Glucagon is often requested during certain surgeries due to various systemic effects. It relaxes gastrointestinal smooth muscle, which includes the sphincter of Oddi. This can help with the passing of bile stones. It also increases myocardial contractility, which can be useful after cardiac surgery or in cases of heart failure. Lastly, it promotes glycogenolysis, which may be used in cases of hypoglycemia.

Dose-response Curve - Descriptive Characteristics

PIES

Potency
Individual variability
Efficacy
Slope

If you're anything like me, your eyes begin to glaze over anytime you hear the words "dose-response curve." But it's something we should know since we give multiple drugs all day. This type of graph charts the dose of a particular drug on one axis and that drug's response on the other. Dose-response curves are differentiated by potency, individual variability, efficacy, and the slope of the curve. So this means there will be differences based on the strength of a drug, how each individual reacts, and how well it produced the desired effect.

Membrane Diffusion – Dependent Factors

Move **T**hat **L**azy **C**rap

Molecular Weight
Thickness of Membrane
Lipid Solubility
Concentration Gradient

The diffusion of a drug across the cell membrane is dependent upon several factors. A substance with a high molecular weight will have a lower rate of diffusion than that a substance with a smaller molecular weight. The thicker the cell membrane, the lower the diffusion rate. The more lipid soluble a substance is, the higher the diffusion rate. Finally, the higher the concentration gradient, the greater the diffusion rate. Maybe this will help you remember:

MORE molecular weight = LOWER diffusion
MORE membrane thickness = LOWER diffusion
MORE lipid solubility = GREATER diffusion
MORE concentration gradient = GREATER diffusion

Intra-arterial Thiopental Injection – Signs and Symptoms

ABC

Arterial vasospasm
Blanching of skin
Cyanosis

Although thiopental is used less these days, it is still utilized in some places and still can show up on tests. If thiopental is accidentally injected into an artery, the patient will experience a few problems. They will likely have intense pain in the arm with arterial vasospasm. You may see distal pulses disappear and blanching of the skin. Finally, the patient could become cyanotic and the site of administration might eventually become gangrenous.

Naloxone – Opioid Actions Easily Reversed

PUN

Pruritus
Urinary retention
Nausea and vomiting

Naloxone – Opioid Actions Reversed with Higher Doses

Reverse **S**andman

Respiratory Depression
Sedation (Profound)

Narcan is a great drug that can help reverse some of the effects from too much opioid. But some of these effects disappear more easily than others. Narcan doesn't have much of a problem taking away the itching, nausea, and urinary retention caused by opioids. However, it has a harder time reversing the profound sedative and respiratory depression effects. These symptoms may require higher doses to achieve the desired effect.

Plasma Cholinesterase – Conditions that Diminish its Activity

PLAY

Pregnancy
Liver disease
Atypical plasma cholinesterase
Young age

Succinylcholine and ester local anesthetics are metabolized by plasma cholinesterase. Therefore, diminishing plasma cholinesterase will prolong the action of these drugs. Keep this in mind when taking care of certain patients. It is diminished during pregnancy and in liver cirrhosis. It is also diminished in the first six months of life and if these patients have atypical plasma cholinesterase.

Non-Depolarizing Muscle Relaxants – Potentiating Drugs

CLAD

Calcium channel blockers
Local anesthetics
Aminoglycoside antibiotics
Dantrolene

Non-depolarizing muscle relaxants may be potentiated by certain medications, making them last longer than they normally would. This is true in the case of calcium channel blockers, local anesthetics, aminoglycoside antibiotics, and dantrolene. Keep this in mind when giving these paralytics to patients on these drugs and adjust the dosage accordingly.

Antimuscarinics – Administration Reasons

BIRDS

Bronchodilation
Increase Heart Rate
Reversal of Cholinergic Crisis
Decrease Airway Secretions
Sedation and Amnesia

Antimuscarinics are anticholinergics that block the muscarinic, rather than nicotinic, acetylcholine receptors. Some of the effects are desirable and some aren't, depending on the patient and the situation. Some of the reasons you might give antimuscarinics include bronchodilation, increase heart rate, reverse cholinergic crisis (atropine), sedation and amnesia (scopolamine), and to decrease airway secretions (antisialagogue effect).

Cholinesterase Inhibitors – Quaternary vs Tertiary

A **PEN** costs a **Quarter**

Pyridostigmine
Edrophonium
Neostigmine

are **Quater**nary ammonium substances, meaning they are charged and have four substituents.

PHYSics is **TER**rifying

Physostigmine

is a **Ter**tiary amine, meaning it is uncharged (so it readily crosses the blood-brain barrier) and has three substituents.

Class I Antiarrhythmics – Uses

SAW

Supraventricular dysrhythmias
Atrial fibrillation
Wolff-Parkinson-White syndrome

Antiarrhythmics are used to treat several abnormal cardiac rhythms and are divided into classes. Class I antiarrhythmics work primarily by blocking the sodium channel. They are often used to treat supraventricular and some ventricular dysrhythmias. They also have the ability to slow the atrial rate, which is helpful for atrial fibrillation. For patients with Wolff-Parkinson-White syndrome, these medications can help to suppress the tachyarrhythmias. Common drugs in this class include lidocaine, flecainide, phenytoin, and procainamide.

Calcium Channel Blockers – Uses

SAVE

Supraventricular tachydysrhythmias
Angina pectoris
Vasospasm
Essential Hypertension

Calcium channel blockers are separated into dihydropyridines and non-dihydropyridines, which are also subclassified into phenylalkylamines and benzothiazepines. They are commonly used to treat supraventricular tachyarrhythmias, hypertension, angina, coronary artery vasospasm, and cerebral artery vasospasm. Examples of dihydropyridines include drugs like amlodipine, nicardipine, and nifedipine. Verapamil is the only phenylalkylamine in use currently, while diltiazem is the only benzothiazepine in use currently.

Protamine – Adverse Effects

SAP

Systemic hypotension
Allergic reactions
Pulmonary hypertension

Protamine is used to reverse heparin by forming a stable complex that neutralizes its anticoagulant activity. The adverse effects from protamine administration are usually related to the histamine release it causes. You may see systemic hypotension, allergic reactions, or pulmonary hypertension. These may be exacerbated if pushed too quickly. Allergic reactions are more common in diabetic patients who take NPH insulin and men who have had a vasectomy.

Conversions

% to mg/mL

If you want to know the concentration of a drug, but all you have is the percent (%), it's simple to figure out how many milligrams (mg) there are per milliliter (mL). Simply move the decimal point to the right by one place. For example:

0.2%: 2 mg/mL
5%: 50 mg/mL

1:100,000 to mcg/mL

A simple shortcut for converting a 1:100,000 solution (or similar) to mcg/mL is to divide 1 million (1,000,000) by the denominator. For example:

1,000,000/100,000: 10 mcg/mL

Anaphylactic Reactions – Hypnotics Likely to Cause

Makes **T**hem **P**uffy

Midazolam
Thiopental
Propofol

Anaphylactic reactions are a cause for extreme concern, and many medications are known to provoke it. Three common hypnotics used in anesthesia are also more likely than others to cause anaphylaxis. Propofol is the most likely hypnotic medication to trigger such a reaction.

Anesthesia Basics

Gas Cylinders – Amount Remaining

The amount remaining in the cylinder can be determined by the reading on the pressure gauge with these 4 gases:

NOAH

Nitrogen
Oxygen
Air
Helium

If gases are in liquid form in the cylinder, then the amount remaining cannot be ascertained simply by reading the pressure gauge. However, nitrogen, oxygen, air, and helium are all gases that are not in liquid form in high pressure cylinders. Therefore, you can determine the amount remaining by reading the pressure gauge.

Orbital Muscles

IS SLIM

Inferior Rectus
Superior Rectus

Superior Oblique
Lateral Rectus
Inferior Oblique
Medial Rectus

Inferior Rectus: look down (Cranial nerve III – oculomotor)
Superior Rectus: look up (Cranial nerve III – oculomotor)

Superior Oblique: look in and down (Cranial nerve IV – trochlear)
Lateral Rectus: look outward (Cranial nerve VI – abducens)
Inferior Oblique: look out and up (Cranial nerve III – oculomotor)
Medial Rectus: look inward (Cranial nerve III – oculomotor)

Aldrete's Scoring System – Criteria

ARCCC

Activity
Respiration
Circulation
Consciousness
Color

The Aldrete's scoring system is used by the post-anesthesia care unit to determine when it's safe to discharge the patient to the next phase. The five criteria that comprise this system include activity, respiration, circulation, consciousness, and color. Each of these is worth 0 to 2 points and patients can be discharged when their score is greater than 8. However, they may be kept longer if the nurses and doctors deem it necessary.

Medical Negligence Action - Elements

Dumb **B**oys **D**on't **C**all

Duty
Breach of Duty
Damage
Cause

If a plaintiff brings forth a medical negligence action, they must prove that duty, breach of duty, damage, and 'cause' all existed in their case. Duty means that a reasonable standard of care was expected. Breach of duty means that this standard was not met in some way. Damage means that physical or emotional injury occurred. Cause means that the damage was caused by the defendant. The damage to the plaintiff must be a direct result of the defendant's action.

MRI Contraindications – Implanted Devices

CAB

Cardiac pacemakers
AICD
Biological pumps

Any object with a high susceptibility to magnetization could place the patient or that object at risk during an MRI. Biological pumps, such as implanted pain pumps and insulin pumps, may get damaged or cause harm to the patient. The same can be said for pacemakers and AICDs, which may convert to asynchronous mode, be deactivated, or get switch damage. MRIs may also be contraindicated in patients with vascular clips, stents, and wire-spiraled endotracheal tubes.

Soda Lime Exhaustion - Indicators

FAITH

Flushed dry skin
Absorbent turns color
Inspired CO2 concentration increases
Tachycardia
Hypertension

When the patient is showing any signs of increased CO2 production, then you might want to take a look at your soda lime canister to see if it needs to be changed. Common signs of soda lime exhaustion include flushed dry skin, tachycardia, and hypertension. The easiest way to tell though, is by looking at your CO2 waveform and the canister itself. If the patient is rebreathing CO2, the absorbent has changed color, and there is a large amount of condensation in the canister, then the soda lime has probably been exhausted. Get a new one!

Awareness During Anesthesia – Increased Risk

PITA (Pain In The Ass)

Provider abuse of anesthetic drugs
Inhalational agent not turned on/empty vaporizer
TIVA not begun or failure of device
Anesthesia discontinued too early

Awareness during anesthesia can be a very scary thing for our patients. One of the most asked questions in the pre-operative area is "how do you know if I'm asleep enough?" Although a rare occurrence, there are some things that may increase the risk of awareness. If the anesthesia provider is abusing the anesthetics, then they may charge some drugs to the patient but never administer them, instead pocketing them for later. The anesthetist may forget to turn on the gas or simply forget to fill the vaporizer. Another problem may occur during a TIVA when gas can't be used. After induction, the IV meds may be forgotten (since the anesthetist is used to turning on the gas, rather than starting a pump). Lastly, anesthesia may be discontinued too early. As the surgery is ending, the anesthetist may cut the gas too early in trying to achieve "the perfect wakeup."

Volatile Anesthetics – Renal Changes

RUG

Renal blood flow
Urine output
Glomerular filtration rate

Volatile anesthetics can affect many body systems in various ways, and the kidneys are no exception. They can cause decreases in renal blood flow, urine output, and glomerular filtration rate. Desflurane may be a better choice in patients with already impaired renal function.

Gamma Amino Butyric Acid Type A (GABA_A) Receptor – Ligand Binding Sites

GABAS **P**ossessive **B**inding **P**laces

G
Anesthetics
Barbiturates
Alcohol
Steroids

Propofol
Benzodiazepines
Picrotoxin

We should all be familiar with the name gamma amino butyric acid (GABA), since it is believed to have much to do with the function of anesthesia. If you look closely, you'll see that five of these sites involve anesthesia. GABA Type A ligand binding sites include anesthetics, barbiturates, alcohol, steroids, Propofol, benzodiazepines, and picrotoxin.

Heat Loss – Causes (Most to Least)

Really **C**over **E**very **C**orner

Radiation >
Convection >
Evaporation >
Conduction

As anesthesia providers, we're responsible for the maintenance of patient temperature, making sure they don't get hypothermic. Therefore, it's important to know how heat is lost so we can figure out ways to stop it. During anesthesia, heat is mostly lost through radiation, which is the transfer of heat from the body to other cooler things nearby. The patient loses heat when the ambient temperature in the operating room is too low. Convection happens when forced air flows over exposed skin and removes heat along with it. Heat is lost by evaporation through use of surgical prep solutions and open cavities in the body. Conduction is when heat gets transferred from the body to a surface it is in contact with, such as the cold operating room bed.

Volatile Inhaled Agents – Trade Names

HF – **H**epatic **F**ailure
EE – **E**vil **E**mpire
IF – **I** **F**arted
DS – **D**ark **S**ide
SU – **S**uck **U**p

Halothane is **F**luothane™
Enflurane is **E**thrane™
Isoflurane is **F**orane™
Desflurane is **S**uprane™
Sevoflurane is **U**ltane™

Nitrous Oxide (N$_2$O) – Side Effects

CACA

Congenital anomalies
Aplastic anemia
CNS toxicity
Abortion (Spontaneous)

As we all know, nitrous oxide isn't without serious side effects. For instance, it is known to cause nausea and can also get trapped in closed air spaces, so should be avoided in certain patients. It may cause spontaneous abortion or congenital anomalies, so avoid or use caution in pregnant patients, particularly during organogenesis. Nitrous oxides could also cause central nervous system toxicity and aplastic anemia. Although it can be a very useful drug, be cautious when administering and make sure you think before you turn that dial.

Anesthetic Brain Uptake – Dependent Factors

Anesthesia **I**s **B**riskly **C**hanging

Alveolar Ventilation
Inspired Concentration
Blood Solubility
Cardiac Output

The uptake of volatile anesthetics by the brain is dependent upon several factors. The higher the alveolar ventilation, the faster the uptake. The more you increase the inspired concentration, the faster the uptake. The more blood soluble a gas is, the slower the uptake, due to the slower rise in alveolar partial pressure. Finally, when a patient has a lower cardiac output, it increases the uptake to the brain.

HIGHER Alveolar ventilation = FASTER uptake
HIGHER Inspired concentration = FASTER uptake
HIGHER Blood solubility = SLOWER uptake
HIGHER Cardiac output = SLOWER uptake

Complications / Disorders

Fluid Overload in the TURP Patient – Late Signs

DASH

Dyspnea
Arrhythmias
Seizures
Hyponatremia (severe)/ **H**ypotension

When a patient is undergoing a TURP procedure, fluid overload is a potential complication due to the large amount of fluid used during surgery. These can lead to several problems, but later signs include shortness of breath, arrhythmias, seizures, hypotension, and severe hyponatremia. Most of the problems arise because of the dilution of the sodium in the body.

Delayed Gastric Emptying – Possible Causes

POOP a **TAD**

Pregnancy
Obesity
Opioids
Pain

Trauma
Anxiety
Diabetes

When your patient has delayed gastric emptying, it puts them at a much higher risk for aspiration and PONV. Therefore, it's important to identify them pre-operatively. Some common causes include obesity, opioid use, pain, anxiety, and trauma. Patients who have been involved in a trauma should be considered NPO only up until the time of the trauma. If they had lunch at 1200, and they get in a car accident at 1500, they should be considered NPO for 3 hours, even if surgery isn't until 2000. The obvious causes for delayed gastric emptying are diabetes and pregnancy. Take caution with these patients.

Carcinoid Syndrome – Overproduced Hormonal Mediators

Some **P**enises **H**ave **B**umpy **K**nots

Serotonin
Prostaglandins
Histamine
Bradykinin
Kallikrein

Carcinoid syndrome happens because of carcinoid tumors, which most often present in the lungs or the digestive tract. It can cause overproduction of several hormonal mediators, including prostaglandins, histamine, bradykinin, and kallikrein. But the hallmark of carcinoid syndrome is serotonin overproduction. These produce several signs and symptoms, such as flushing and diarrhea. If the tumors are present in the lungs, you may also see dyspnea, chest pain, wheezing, or weight gain. If the tumors are present in the digestive tract, you could see abdominal pain, rectal pain and bleeding, bowel obstruction, or nausea.

Myotonic Dystrophy – Anesthetic Concerns

CRAP

Cardiomyopathy
Respiratory muscle weakness
Aspiration of gastric contents
Potential for abnormal responses to anesthetic drugs

Myotonic dystrophy is an inherited disorder and causes progressive muscle weakness. This creates cause for concern for the anesthetist in a variety of ways. These patients may present with arrhythmias, cardiomyopathy, and congestive heart failure. They may also have respiratory muscle weakness, so be cautious when using drugs that may cause respiratory depression. Myotonic dystrophy may cause decreased GI motility and lower esophageal sphincter tone, putting them at risk for aspiration. You may want to consider rapid sequence. You should also keep in mind that the reactions to anesthetic medications may not be as expected.

TURP – Glycine Side Effects

ANTHEM

Ammonia toxicity
Nausea and vomiting
Transient blindness
Headache
ECG changes
Myocardial depression

Transurethral resection of the prostate (TURP) involves the use of an irrigating agent, each with its own set of complications. If the surgeon uses glycine, it may lead to ammonia toxicity, nausea and vomiting, headache, ectopy, myocardial depression, and blindness (that typically resolves). The patient may also experience loss of light and accommodation reflexes. This is all in addition to the already present risk of fluid overload. Having the patient awake, using regional anesthesia, may help identify some of these symptoms earlier, allowing for quicker treatment.

Malignant Hyperthermia – Complications After it's Controlled

Rx MEDS

Recurrence

Myoglobinuric renal failure
Electrolyte abnormalities
Disseminated intravascular coagulation (DIC)
Skeletal muscle weakness

Malignant hyperthermia is a very dangerous potential complication of general anesthesia. If the patient is lucky enough to survive the initial attack, there are still several hurdles they will encounter before they are out of the woods. Recurrence of MH is a very strong possibility. The patient may also have myoglobinuric renal failure due to rhabdomyolysis, electrolyte abnormalities, skeletal muscle weakness, and DIC. All of this is caused by the calcium buildup in the skeletal muscle. Assuming Dantrolene was given, this should be continued as recommended in the post-operative period.

Malignant Hyperthermia – Active Cooling Methods

Ice **C**old **L**ife **S**upport

Intravenous normal saline
Cardiopulmonary bypass (in severe cases)
Lavage
Surface cooling

Malignant hyperthermia is a rare problem that anesthetists pray they will never have to come across. However, if it does happen, there are ways you can help actively cool the patient while giving the dantrolene. Chilled normal saline can be given intravenously. Lavage is also an option, using the orogastric route, urinary bladder, or into any open cavities. Ice packs should be placed at the patient's groin, neck, and axilla. Forced-air blankets that blow cold can also be implemented. In severe cases, cardiopulmonary bypass may be necessary to allow for cooling.

Mandibular Hypoplasia – Associated Congenital Diseases

PG Television

Pierre Robin Syndrome
Goldenhar Syndrome
Treacher Collins Syndrome

Mandibular hypoplasia is a condition that often causes an abnormal airway, making it more difficult to intubate. Three examples of congenital mandibular hypoplasia include Pierre Robin Syndrome, Goldenhar Syndrome, and Treacher Collins Syndrome. Although they are considered a difficult airway, these patients are often intubated after they go to sleep. Awake fiber optic intubation can be used, but it may do more harm than good. It can cause severe damage to the upper airway and they are still at risk for aspiration.

Chronic Alcoholics - Hematologic Abnormalities

Apparent **L**iver **T**rouble

Anemia
Leukopenia
Thrombocytopenia

Chronic alcoholics slowly, but surely, cause damage their liver that will usually kill them eventually if they don't stop drinking. This liver damage can lead to several hematologic abnormalities, including anemia, leukopenia, and thrombocytopenia. These patients are at a higher risk for bleeding, so keep that in mind during high risk surgeries. Medications that can worsen the liver damage should be avoided unless the benefits outweigh the risks.

Bladder Perforation – Signs and Symptoms

BAD HANDS

Bradycardia
Anxiety
Diaphoresis

Hypotension/Hiccups
Abdominal pain
Nausea
Dyspnea
Shoulder pain

Bladder perforation typically happens for 2 reasons: either it gets way overdistended or something punctures it. For example, in a TURP procedure, the irrigation fluid may cause too much pressure until the bladder wall can no longer hold. It may also happen if the surgeon accidentally hits the bladder with the resectoscope.

Bladder perforation may be intraperitoneal, extraperitoneal, or both. Intraperitoneal perforation usually happens in the dome of the bladder and may cause pain in the precordial area, shoulder, upper abdomen, or neck. Extraperitoneal perforation usually happens in the base of the bladder and may cause lower abdominal distention and pain in the inguinal, periumbilical, or suprapubic areas. Patients with bladder perforation may also have bradycardia, anxiety, diaphoresis, hypotension, hiccups, nausea, and shortness of breath.

Lower Esophageal Sphincter Tone – Factors That Decrease

G SHOP

Glucagon

Secretin
Hiatal hernia
Obesity
Pregnancy

Lower esophageal sphincter tone is important because it helps prevent stomach contents from going up back into the esophagus. When the LES tone is lower, stomach contents are much more likely to re-enter the esophagus. This is important for us to know in anesthesia because a decreased LES tone greatly increases the risk for aspiration. You may want to consider doing a rapid sequence induction in these patients. Lower esophageal sphincter tone is decreased by many things, including pregnancy, obesity, hiatal hernia, secretin, and glucagon.

Glucose-6-phosphate-dehydrogenase (G6PDH) Deficiency – Drugs to Avoid

MD NAPS

Methylene blue
Doxorubicin

Nitroprusside
Aspirin
Penicillin/**P**rilocaine
Streptomycin/**S**ulfonamides

Glucose-6-phosphate-dehydrogenase (G6PDH) deficiency causes the breakdown of red blood cells. Although patients with this disorder often don't have any symptoms, it is not uncommon for them to experience malaise, dyspnea, dark urine, and jaundice. Medications that may trigger an episode should be avoided if possible. Some of these include methylene blue, doxorubicin, nitroprusside, aspirin, penicillin, prilocaine, streptomycin, and sulfonamides.

Duchenne Muscular Dystrophy – Anesthetic Concerns

CURDS

Cardiac arrest upon induction
Unpredictable susceptibility to malignant hyperthermia
Retention of pulmonary secretions
Delayed gastric emptying
Succinylcholine-induced hyperkalemia

Duchenne muscular dystrophy is a progressive disorder that causes the muscles to become weaker as time goes by. It is first diagnosed in childhood and affects primarily males. Because of the nature of the disease, we must be vigilant as anesthesia providers in anticipating certain complications. These patients have weakened heart muscle, so it is possible for them to go into cardiac arrest during the stress of induction. Also, because it is a muscular disorder, they may be more susceptible to malignant hyperthermia. They might have delayed gastric emptying and retention of pulmonary secretions, and they may be more difficult to extubate due to weakened breathing muscles. Be aware of the possibility of increased potassium after succinylcholine administration, even more so than the usual response.

Syndrome of Inappropriate ADH Secretion (SIADH) – Causes

CHIP

Carcinoma of the lung
Hypothyroidism
Intracranial tumors
Porphyria

In Syndrome of Inappropriate ADH Secretion (SIADH), too much ADH is being released into the body, causing too much fluid to be retained. This leads to dilution of sodium and resultant hyponatremia. Common causes include lung cancer or disease, hypothyroidism, brain tumors, and porphyria. The most common reason for SIADH is intracranial tumors. The hyponatremia and fluid overload in these patients may cause nausea, muscle weakness, tremors, shortness of breath, confusion, seizures, coma, and even death if left untreated.

Syndrome of Inappropriate ADH Secretion - Treatment

CHAR

Correct underlying cause
Hyperosmotic saline
Antagonize the effects of ADH
Restrict water intake

In Syndrome of Inappropriate ADH Secretion (SIADH), too much ADH is being released into the body, causing too much fluid to be retained. This leads to dilution of sodium and resultant hyponatremia. Common causes include lung cancer or disease, hypothyroidism, brain tumors, and porphyria. The hyponatremia and fluid overload in these patients may cause nausea, muscle weakness, tremors, shortness of breath, confusion, seizures, coma, and even death. Treatment should be first directed at correcting the underlying problem. Otherwise, you'll end up just chasing the symptoms. You can also give hyperosmotic saline (can be given with or without diuretics), restrict the intake of water, and give demecolcine. Demecolcine can antagonize the ADH effects on the renal tubule.

Diabetic Autonomic Neuropathy – Anesthetic Concerns

POG

Painless myocardial infarction
Orthostatic hypotension
Gastroparesis

Diabetic autonomic neuropathy affects the nervous system throughout the body, typically caused by poor glucose control. The nerves become damaged and are unable to function properly. These patients often have difficulty sensing feeling in their feet and may have poor eyesight. Gastroparesis is common, and the delayed gastric emptying puts them at a greater risk for aspiration. They may also be more likely to have silent heart attacks and orthostatic hypotension. Be ready with vasopressors, as they tend to need more support than patients without autonomic neuropathy.

Pheochromocytoma – Signs and Symptoms

Hormone-**D**ischarging **T**umor

Hypertension/**H**eadache
Diaphoresis
Tachycardia

A pheochromocytoma is a tumor located on the adrenal gland, specifically arising from the chromaffin cells. It stores and is capable of secreting catecholamines, sometimes in very large amounts. This causes hypertension, tachycardia, and diaphoresis. These patients often complain of a headache. The tumor is usually only located on one adrenal gland or the other, but it is seen bilaterally in some cases. Nonselective beta blockers should be avoided without proper alpha blockade also. Doing so could leave the vasoconstriction of alpha receptors unopposed without the beta-2 vasodilation.

Chronic Renal Failure - Pathophysiological Consequences

(in addition to electrolyte disturbances)

CHAMPS

Coagulopathies
Hypertension
Anemia
Metabolic acidosis
Pruritus
Susceptibility to infection

We all know about the electrolyte disturbances that may be present in patients with chronic renal failure. But we should also keep in mind the other problems that may arise from this condition. These patients are usually fluid overloaded and unable to clear a lot of the toxins that are normally excreted in the urine. Coagulopathies, high blood pressure, anemia, and pruritus are not uncommon. They are also more susceptible to infections. Don't forget about the metabolic acidosis that may be caused by the fluid and electrolyte shifts.

Complex Regional Pain Syndrome (CRPS) – Signs and Symptoms

ASSHAT

Active and Passive Motor Disorders
Sympathetic Dysfunction
Spontaneous Pain
Hyperalgia
Allodynia
Trophic, Sudomotor, Vasomotor Abnormalities

Complex Regional Pain Syndrome (CRPS) is a group of conditions that cause pain and swelling, usually starting in an arm or leg. It may start after some sort of trauma or injury and may affect the entire body in some patients. Some of the signs and symptoms to remember include active and passive motor disorders, hyperalgesia, and allodynia. These patients can also have sympathetic dysfunction, which may be seen as swelling and cyanosis. Pain can present spontaneously, without anything bringing it on. They may also have trophic, vasomotor and sudomotor (sweat gland) abnormalities. It is considered Type I CRPS if there is no evidence of nerve damage to the limb, while it is considered Type II if there is evidence of nerve damage in the limb.

Prune-belly Syndrome – Congenital Anomalies

Unstable **A**bdominal **C**ondition

Urinary tract abnormalities
Absent abdominal wall muscles
Cryptorchidism

Prune-belly syndrome is a rare inherited disorder that causes problems with the urinary system. This condition can sometimes create areas of wrinkled skin on the stomach, which is where it gets its name. There are no associated problems with the gastrointestinal system. Instead, it is known for a triad of anomalies, including undescended testes (cryptorchidism), absent or partially absent abdominal wall muscles, and urinary tract abnormalities. These patients can also have club foot, ventricular septal defect, frequent UTIs, and musculoskeletal abnormalities.

Burns – Fluid Resuscitation (PA Cath Parameters)

Cool **M**o **F**os

Cardiac output
Mixed venous oxygen tension
Filling pressures

After a burn injury, administration of fluids is paramount in the initial phase. Fluids should be titrated according to specific goals, as outlined in formulas such as the Parke or modified Brooke. These goals can be monitored easily by using a pulmonary artery catheter. Fluid resuscitation can be shown to be adequate by reaching an acceptable cardiac output, mixed venous oxygen tension, and filling pressures.

Monitoring and Equipment

Medical Gas Lines - Common Contaminants

B WORM

Bacteria

Water
Oil
Residual sterilizing solutions.
Matter

Although medical gas lines are inspected for safety and contaminants, many things are often missed, due to inexperience and lack of expertise. Water is the most common contaminant, but there has also been reports of oil, bacteria, and particulate matter, such as dirt, sand, gravel, and dust. Sterilizing solutions have also been found, left as residual from previous use. These contaminants often enter during the initial construction of the pipelines. Anesthesia providers should make themselves aware of the safety code and be able to give input during construction. If already contaminated, the pipelines should be cleaned or purged.

Modern Vaporizers – Hazards

LOITER

Leaks
Overfilling with agent
Incorrect agent administration
Tipping
Reliance on breath-by-breath gas analysis

Over the years, anesthesia vaporizers have undergone many changes and technological advancements to improve the way we deliver care. But even today, there are still some hazards that they can present. Vaporizers can still leak and have electronic failures. There is nothing to prevent you from overfilling them with agents. It may be possible to fill certain ones with the wrong agent still, and there is also a heavy reliance now on breath-by-breath gas analysis, rather than preventative maintenance to keep problems from happening.

Proportion-Limiting Systems – Conditions That Can "Fool" Them

WILD

Wrong supply gas
Inert gas administration
Leaks downstream
Defective pneumatics or mechanics
Dilution of inspired oxygen concentration

In anesthesia workstations equipped with proportioning systems, hypoxic gas mixtures may be delivered in certain conditions. This includes the wrong supply gas, inert gas administration, downstream leaks, defective mechanics/pneumatics, or dilution of inspired oxygen concentration by volatile anesthetics.

Required Monitors on the Anesthesia Workstation

BIO HEAP

Blood pressure
Inspired Oxygen
Oxygen Supply Failure Alarm

Hypoxic guard system
Electrocardiogram (ECG)
Anesthetic Vapor Concentration
Pulse Oximetry

BIO HEAP is a good way to remember the basic required monitors on an anesthesia workstation. Blood pressure monitoring is a must, as is an inspired oxygen alarm, which must alarm within 30 seconds after the oxygen being delivered goes under 18%. There has to be an oxygen supply failure alarm and a hypoxic guard system that stops you from going under 21% oxygen when using nitrous. Lastly, the anesthesia workstation must have ecg monitoring, pulse oximetry, and anesthesia vapor concentration.

Regional Anesthesia

Stellate Ganglion Blockade (Horner's Syndrome) - Signs and Symptoms

FACES

Flushing
Anhidrosis
Congestion
Eyes
Skin temperature increased

A stellate ganglion block is done to blunt the sympathetic system on the ipsilateral side of the arm and the face. Horner's syndrome indicates that a successful blockade has occurred. Signs and symptoms of Horner's Syndrome include facial and arm flushing (vasodilation), anhidrosis (lack of sweating), nasal congestion, ptosis, miosis, and increased skin temperature.

Neuraxial Block – Dyspnea Causes

PHAT

Position
Hypotension
Abdominal and intercostal muscles blockade
Thoracic proprioception blunting

During a spinal or epidural, dyspnea is a fairly common complication. There may be several possible causes for this, but the most common is hypotension. This is because the decreased blood pressure causes hypoperfusion in the brainstem. So if someone complains of shortness of breath after a neuraxial block, the first thought should be low blood pressure. However, it can also be caused by other things, such as simple positioning, when the abdominal contents are pressing up against the diaphragm. Dyspnea may also be due to a partial block of the abdominal and intercostal muscles. Finally, there may also be blunting of thoracic proprioception, in which patients have difficulty "feeling" the chest wall moving while taking a breath.

Spinal and Epidural Opioids – Side Effects

LINEUPS

Late respiratory depression
Ileus
Nausea and vomiting
Early respiratory depression
Urinary retention
Pruritus
Sedation

Giving opioids via epidural or spinal is not without potential side effects and complications. The thing you might worry about the most is delayed respiratory depression. But, don't forget about nausea, vomiting, itching, sedation, urinary retention, and eventual ileus down the road. Early respiratory depression is one of the least likely complications to arise.

High Spinal Anesthesia – Signs and Symptoms

HAND

Hypotension
Apnea
Nausea and vomiting
Dyspnea

A high spinal happens when the amount of medication is overestimated for the patient, resulting in a block above the desired level (usually T4). The reaction can vary in severity depending on how high it goes. Some common signs and symptoms include hypotension, shortness of breath, nausea, vomiting, and even respiratory failure. If it goes high enough, it could become a total spinal, causing the patient to lose consciousness. Cardiac arrest and death could follow if not dealt with quickly.

Retrobulbar Block – Desired Effects

AAA

Akinesia of the eye
Anesthesia of the eye
Abolishment of the oculo-cardiac reflex

The retrobulbar space is the area that is behind the globe of the eye. A retrobulbar block is done for eye surgeries, most often for cataract correction. A desired block will produce akinesia of the extraocular muscles, abolishment of the oculo-cardiac reflex, and anesthesia of the conjunctiva, cornea, and uvea.

Surgical Procedures

Mediastinoscopy - Relative Contraindications

CATS

Cerebrovascular disease
Aortic aneurysm (thoracic)
Tracheal deviation
Superior vena cava obstruction

Mediastinoscopy is typically done to get lymph node biopsies to help stage lung cancer. It may also be done to aid in the diagnosis of other conditions like lymphoma or sarcoidosis. Relative contraindications include cerebrovascular disease, thoracic aortic aneurysm, tracheal deviation, and SVC obstruction. If the benefits outweigh the risks, then proceed with great caution in these cases. You don't want to end up with a complication like a stroke or aneurysm rupture.

LeFort III Fracture – Important Considerations

TIP

Tracheostomy
Intubation
Positioning

A Lefort III fracture is when all of the facial bones separate away from the cranial base, along with fractures of zygoma, nasal, and maxilla bones. These patients often have very limited mouth opening and instability of the facial structures, making intubation a challenge. After positioning optimally, consider an awake fiberoptic intubation. Another option is to go straight to a tracheostomy under local only anesthesia. Cricothyrotomy should be anticipated, but only done in case of emergency.

Mediastinoscopy – Vessels That Can Be Compressed

SIC

Subclavian Arteries
Innominate Artery
Carotid Arteries

Mediastinoscopy is typically done to get lymph node biopsies to help stage lung cancer. It may also be done to aid in the diagnosis of other conditions like lymphoma or sarcoidosis. During this procedure, the subclavian arteries, carotid arteries, and the innominate artery may be compressed. If the innominate artery is compressed, it will cause reduced blood flow through the right carotid and right subclavian arteries. It can also cause a decrease in cerebral perfusion, as can direct compression of the carotid arteries, especially in patients with cerebral vascular disease. If the right subclavian artery is directly or indirectly compressed, it will decrease the pressure and pulse in the right arm. It might be a good idea to place the pulse ox on the right hand to monitor for this.

Strabismus Repair – Anesthetic Concerns

COMP

Cardiovascular effects of ocular medications
Oculo-cardiac reflex
Malignant hyperthermia
Postoperative nausea and vomiting

Strabismus repair involves working on the extraocular muscles to correct the underlying problem. But a seemingly simple surgery like this isn't quite so simple when you consider the possible complications. Since the surgeon will be working within the eye, the oculo-cardiac reflex is very much in play (remember the 'five and dime' mnemonic, involving the 5_{th} and 10_{th} cranial nerves). So watch out for bradycardia and nausea and vomiting. You should also be aware of the cardiovascular effects many of the ocular medications have, including CHF and arrhythmias. Patients with strabismus are more likely to have an underlying myopathy, therefore putting them at a greater chance of malignant hyperthermia happening. Stay away from succinylcholine in these patients (to avoid MH and increased intraocular pressure) and consider TIVA (which will also help with the PONV).

Radical Neck Dissection - Intraoperative Complications

BAM

Baroreceptors
Air embolism
Mainstem

Radical neck dissections are done to treat cancers or to prevent the spread of certain cancers. There are a number of possible complications, including but not limited to, baroreceptor compression, air embolism, and inadvertent mainstem intubation. When the baroreceptors are stimulated, the baroreceptor reflex is often initiated, causing bradycardia and hypotension. Because of positioning and manipulation of the head and neck, the endotracheal tube may migrate downward into the mainstem bronchus. This can be monitored for by checking bilateral breath sounds, peak inspiratory pressures, and the CO_2 waveform.

Pathophysiology

Oxyhemoglobin Dissociation Curve - Rightward Shift Causes

2 TAPS

Increased **2**,3-DPG
Increased **T**emperature
Increased (**A**cidity) H+ concentration (decreased pH)
Increased **P**artial pressure of CO_2
Sickle cell disease

When the oxyhemoglobin dissociation curve shifts leftward, the hemoglobin tends to hold on to the oxygen more tightly. When it shifts rightward, the hemoglobin tends to release more oxygen to the tissues. A rightward shift is caused by increased temperature, acidity, partial pressure of carbon dioxide, and 2,3 DPG. It is also caused by sickle cell disease. Try to remember that when metabolism is increased, the curve shifts more to the right. In opposite conditions, it shifts to the left.

Adrenal Medulla – Catecholamines Secreted

END

Epinephrine
Norepinephrine
Dopamine

The adrenal medulla is controlled by the sympathetic nervous system and the hormones secreted by it create the "flight or fight" response. The two main catecholamines secreted are epinephrine and norepinephrine, but also dopamine in smaller amounts.

Natriuretic Peptides

CUBA

CNP (C-Type)
Urodilatin
BNP (Brain/B-Type)
ANP (Atrial/A-Type)

Peptides that cause the kidneys to excrete sodium (natriuresis) are called natriuretic peptides. ANP gets released from atrial muscle when the local walls stretch and when there is increased atrial volume. BNP gets released when ventricular muscle is distended. CNP gets released from the endothelium of major vessels in response to stress and other stimuli. Urodilatin is produced in the lower urinary tract and is excreted when mean arterial pressure (MAP) is increased or blood volume is increased. Natriuretic receptor-A binds ANP and BNP, while natriuretic receptor-B binds CNP.

Immunoglobulins

GAMED

Ig**G**
Ig**A**
Ig**M**
Ig**E**
Ig**D**

Immunoglobulins are basically antibodies that are able to recognize certain antigens, bind to them, and help to destroy them. IgG is found in all fluids in the body and is the most common type, making up around 75% of all serum antibodies. IgA is found mostly in mucous membranes, such as saliva, tears, and respiratory and gastrointestinal tracts. IgM is in the blood and lymph and is the first attacker of an infection. IgE is located in the skin, mucous membranes, and lungs. It is produced when there is an allergen, creating an allergic reaction. Finally, IgD is located in the blood in small amounts and is also co-expressed with IgM.

Signal Transduction Systems - Components

PEERS

Protein
Enzyme
External Signal
Receptor
Second Messenger

Signal transduction is the transfer of signals from the outside of a cell to the inside through its membrane. In this type of system, the first messengers (ligands) are external signals. Primary effectors are activated by the receptors, which are called signal transducers. An enzyme gets coupled to the receptor by a protein. The second messenger is an intracellular chemical that is promoted by an enzyme. The secondary effectors are activated by the second messengers.

That's it! Keep these mnemonics for reference later, and try to come up with some on your own. The process of creating them helps to solidify them even more in your memory. I hope you enjoyed the book, and I wish you the best on your future career as a nurse anesthetist. Don't forget to pick up a copy of another helpful book, Survive CRNA School, available as an e-book or hard copy on Amazon and other booksellers.